THE LOW FODMAP DIET COOKBOOK FOR BEGINNERS

NATALIE BROWN

Copyright ©2023.

TABLE OF CONTENTS

FOREWORD

Sarah had been suffering from digestive issues for years, and she had tried just about every diet out there. When she heard about the Low FODMAP diet, she was intrigued and decided to give it a try.

She quickly realized the benefits of the diet and was able to reduce her symptoms significantly. She also found that she was able to enjoy food again, something she hadn't been able to do in a long time.

Desperate to share her newfound knowledge with others, she decided to compile all the best recipes she could find into one easy-to-use book. She reached out to friends, family, and even strangers online to get their favorite recipes, and she spent hours researching and testing different recipes to make sure they were Low FODMAP-friendly.

Finally, she was able to put together a comprehensive collection of delicious recipes that everyone could enjoy. She was excited to share her book with the world, and she was surprised to find that it quickly became a hit.

People from all over the world started writing in or leaving comments praising Sarah's book and how it had helped them. Sarah was elated; she had found a new passion in helping others, and she found true joy in knowing that her work was making a difference in people's lives.

The Low FODMAP diet had changed Sarah's life, and now she was able to pass on the same benefits to others. She was thankful for the opportunity to share her knowledge and help others find relief from their digestive issues.

WHAT ARE FODMAPS?

FODMAPs are short-chain carbohydrates and sugar alcohols that are poorly digested by the body. They ferment in the large intestine (bowel) during digestion, drawing in water and producing carbon dioxide, hydrogen, and methane gas that causes the intestine to expand. This causes GI symptoms such as bloating and pain that are common in disorders like IBS.

FODMAPs are in some foods naturally or as additives. They include fructose (in fruits and vegetables), fructans (like fructose, found in some vegetables and grains), lactose (dairy), Galatians (legumes), and polyols (artificial sweeteners).

These foods are not necessarily unhealthy products. Some of them contain fructans, inulin, and galactooligosaccharides (GOS), which are healthy prebiotics that helps stimulate the growth of beneficial gut bacteria. Many of them are otherwise good for you, but in certain people, eating or drinking them causes gastrointestinal symptoms.

INTRODUCTION TO LOW FODMAP DIET

FODMAP foods are foods that contain certain types of carbohydrates. They include sugars that can cause symptoms in the digestive systems of susceptible individuals. Studies have shown eating a diet low in FODMAP-containing foods may reduce symptoms of irritable bowel syndrome and other gastrointestinal conditions.

FODMAP stands for *"fermentable oligosaccharides, disaccharides, monosaccharides, and polyols."* Low FODMAP foods are low in these substances.

Irritable bowel syndrome (IBS) is a gastrointestinal disorder that affects 10–15% of adults in the United States, although only 5–7% of adults have received a diagnosis, according to the American College of Gastroenterology. It involves gastrointestinal symptoms, including bloating, diarrhea, and constipation.

The low FODMAP diet may also benefit with inflammatory bowel disease, which includes Crohn's disease and ulcerative colitis. A 2020 studyTrusted Source found, for example, that the diet had a favorable impact on symptoms in people with Crohn's disease. It may help those with celiac disease.

WHAT IS A LOW FODMAP DIET?

A team of researchers from Monash University in Melbourne, Australia, developed The Low FODMAP Diet. The group was the first to prove that low FODMAP diets improved IBS symptoms.

The diet plan classifies FODMAP foods as high and low. It recommends that people with IBS avoid high FODMAP foods and choose low FODMAP foods as their daily staples.

It is important to note that serving sizes can also change how well a person tolerates a specific food. For example, having a large amount of a low FODMAP food could turn it into a high FODMAP food.

Originally, the diet was somewhat restrictive, raising concerns about nutritional deficiencies and disordered eating. Many dietitians now take the approach of a FODMAP-gentle rather than a FOPMAP-free diet. Experts recommend working with a dietitian to avoid both over-restriction and under-restriction.

FOODS TO EAT AND NOT EAT

Protein foods such as meats, poultry, and fish are naturally free of FODMAPs. Some processed and marinated meats may contain high FODMAP ingredients, such as garlic and onion, but not all meat products contain these ingredients. People should discuss their choices with a dietitian.

Low FODMAP foods, which people can eat more liberally than medium and high FODMAP foods, include:

- Vegetables: Lettuces, carrot, chives, fennel, eggplant, broccoli (heads or whole), zucchini, green beans, and baby spinach.
- Fruits: Strawberries, pineapple, grapes, oranges, cucumbers, and kiwifruit.
- Proteins: Chicken, beef, turkey, cold cuts, lamb, tofu, and eggs.
- Fish: Crab, lobster, salmon, tuna, and shrimp.
- Fats: Oils, pumpkin seeds, butter, peanuts, macadamias, and walnuts.

- Starches, cereals, and grains: Potatoes, amaranth, quinoa, brown rice, tortilla chips, and popcorn.

HIGH FODMAP FOODS TO AVOID OR LIMIT INCLUDE:

- Vegetables: Garlic, asparagus, onions, mushrooms, beans, shallots, and scallions.
- Fruits: Blackberries, watermelon, prunes, peaches, dates, and avocados.
- Meats: Breaded meats, battered meats, and meats served with garlic or onion-based sauces and fillings.
- Fish: Breaded fish, battered fish, and fish served with garlic or onion-based sauces.
- Fats: Almonds, cashews, pistachios, and avocados.
- Starches, cereals, and grains: Beans, lentils, wheat and gluten-based bread, rye, muffins, pastries, and pasta.

Knowing the difference between high and low FODMAP foods can make it easier for a person to incorporate them into a diet. Both categories contain a wide range of food groups.

It is essential to talk with a doctor or dietitian before starting a low FODMAP diet. Doctors do not typically recommend this diet plan for long-term use, as it eliminates some essential, nutrient-rich foods.

Many foods high or moderate in FODMAPs contain a number of nutrients, including vitamins, minerals, and prebiotics, which are food components that support healthy gut bacteria.

Symptoms that may improve after following the diet include:

- abdominal pain
- bloating
- diarrhea

BENEFITS OF A LOW-FODMAP DIET

Many people with IBS who use the low-FODMAP diet say it helps them. It may allow you to:

- Have fewer digestive symptoms, like gas, bloating, diarrhea, and constipation
- Manage your IBS symptoms without taking medicine
- Improve your quality of life

HOW DOES A FODMAP DIET WORK?

It is important to note that low FODMAP diets are restrictive and should be temporary, lasting only 4–6 weeks. They aim to identify whether specific foods trigger symptoms.

A low FODMAP diet involves three phases. Monash University, which first proposed the diet, describes them as follows:

- **Step 1:**
  Low FODMAP: In this phase, the person swaps all high FODMAP foods for low FODMAP options for 2–6 weeks. Some people call this the elimination phase, but Monash stresses that it is a case of substitution rather than elimination.
- **Step 2:**
  Reintroduction: Under the guidance of a registered dietitian, the person starts reintroducing FODMAP foods into their diet one at a time. This can help identify which foods trigger symptoms. This phase lasts around 6–8 weeks.

- **Step 3:**

  Personalization: Also known as the maintenance phase, this involves returning to a regular diet as far as possible, limiting only the FODMAP foods that cause IBS symptoms. Eventually, some people may be able to incorporate all or most FODMAPs back into their diet without symptoms.

It is essential to reintroduce foods to see if they cause symptoms, because the aim of the diet is to eliminate only those foods that are troublesome.

2 WEEKS MEAL PLAN FOR LOW FOD MAP DIET

Day 1

- Breakfast: Overnight oats with chia seeds
- Lunch: Kale and quinoa salad
- Dinner: Roasted vegetables and quinoa

Day 2

- Breakfast: Egg and vegetable scramble
- Lunch: Zucchini noodles with pesto
- Dinner: Sweet potato and black bean tacos

Day 3

- Breakfast: Protein smoothie
- Lunch: Avocado toast
- Dinner: Baked salmon with steamed vegetables

Day 4

- Breakfast: Oatmeal with berries
- Lunch: Veggie wrap with hummus
- Dinner: Vegetable stir-fry with brown rice

Day 5

- Breakfast: Yogurt and fruit
- Lunch: Lentil soup
- Dinner: Curried chickpeas and roasted cauliflower

Day 6

- Breakfast: Coconut chia pudding
- Lunch: Grilled chicken salad
- Dinner: Roasted portobello mushrooms with quinoa

Day 7

- Breakfast: Egg and avocado toast
- Lunch: Lentil and vegetable salad
- Dinner: Baked fish with roasted vegetables

Day 8

- Breakfast: Protein smoothie
- Lunch: Veggie wrap with hummus
- Dinner: Chickpea and vegetable curry

Day 9

- Breakfast: Overnight oats with chia seeds
- Lunch: Kale and quinoa salad
- Dinner: Baked salmon with steamed vegetables

Day 10

- Breakfast: Oatmeal with berries
- Lunch: Avocado toast
- Dinner: Vegetable stir-fry with brown rice

Day 11

- Breakfast: Protein smoothie
- Lunch: Lentil soup
- Dinner: Curried chickpeas and roasted cauliflower

Day 12

- Breakfast: Coconut chia pudding
- Lunch: Grilled chicken salad
- Dinner: Roasted portobello mushrooms with quinoa

Day 13

- Breakfast: Egg and avocado toast
- Lunch: Lentil and vegetable salad
- Dinner: Baked fish with roasted vegetables

Day 14

- Breakfast: Yogurt and fruit
- Lunch: Veggie wrap with hummus
- Dinner: Chickpea and vegetable curry

FODMAP DIET RECIPES

VEGAN LOW FODMAP AVOCADO GREEN GODDESS

VEGGIE SANDWICH

INGREDIENTS:

- 2 slices LOFO bread of choice
- ¼ cup (60 ml) Vegan Low FODMAP Avocado Green Goddess Dressing
- ¾ cup (30 g) alfalfa sprouts
- Several leaves of fresh baby arugula
- 1 Persian cucumber, end trimmed, cut into broad ribbons (I use a cheese planer or vegetable peeler)
- 1 slice vegan cheddar cheese, optional

INSTRUCTIONS

1. Slather the Vegan Low FODMAP Avocado Green Goddess Dressing on the bread slices, then layer up with cheese, if using, sprouts, arugula and slices of cucumber.
2. Sandwich is ready to serve or maybe be wrapped in plastic wrap and refrigerated overnight.

FODY'S BAKED HONEY BBQ CHICKEN WINGS

INGREDIENTS:

- 3 lb. chicken wings (about 24 separated pieces)
- 2 Tbsp
- Fody's Shallot Olive Oil
- ¾ cup
- Fody's Original BBQ Sauce
- 1 Tbsp clover honey
- Salt, to taste
- Black pepper, to taste

INSTRUCTIONS

1. Preheat your oven to 400 degrees and line a rimmed baking sheet with parchment paper. Then place a large wire rack on top of the parchment.
2. Next place your chicken wings in a bowl and toss them in your olive oil. Spray the wire rack with non-stick cooking spray and place your chicken wings on the rack. Season them with salt and pepper (be very

generous with the pepper) and bake for 30-35 minutes.

3. While the wings are cooking, heat your low FODMAP bbq sauce and honey in a small pot over medium low heat. (Stir occasionally to make sure the honey is fully mixed in.)

4. Once the baked chicken wings are done, brush them with your sauce and place them back in the oven for 5 minutes. (You can also broil the wings at this point to get them crispier. Just keep checking them to make sure they don't burn. They might not take the whole 5 minutes.)

5. Serve immediately.

LOW FODMAP BANANA NUT OATMEAL MUFFINS

INGREDIENTS

- 2 large ripe bananas
- 2 1/2 cups quick oats (gluten-free if needed)
- 1 1/2 cups lactose-free milk (almond milk for dairy-free)
- 1/4 cup pure maple syrup
- 1 large egg, lightly beaten

- 2 tablespoons canola oil
- 1 teaspoon baking powder
- 1 1/2 teaspoons ground cinnamon
- 1 teaspoon vanilla extract
- 1/4 teaspoon salt
- 1/2 cup chopped walnuts
- 1/4 cup Enjoy Life Dairy-Free Mini Chocolate Chips (or finely chopped dark chocolate)

INSTRUCTIONS

1. Heat oven to 350 degrees F and coat a 12-count non-stick muffin tin with cooking spray.
2. In a large bowl, mash the bananas with a fork. Add the oats and milk. Stir until evenly combined. Let soak about 5 to 10 minutes, or until most of the liquid is absorbed.
3. To the oat mixture, add the maple syrup, egg, canola oil, baking powder, cinnamon, vanilla and salt. Stir until thoroughly combined. Stir in the walnuts and chocolate or chocolate chips.
4. Fill each muffin cup with approximately 1/3 cup of the batter. Bake for 30 to 35 minutes or until lightly browned and tops spring back

when lightly touched in the middle on top. Cool in pan for 10 minutes, then remove to cooling rack.

5. Refrigerate leftover muffins for up to 2 days or freeze for up to 3 months in an airtight, resealable bag.

LOW FODMAP CHICKEN PARMESAN WITH ROASTED VEGETABLE TOMATO SAUCE

INGREDIENTS

- 1 small eggplant, diced small
- 1 zucchini, diced small
- 1 red or yellow bell pepper, diced small
- 2 tbsp olive oil
- Salt & pepper
- 1 plain sausage (just salt & pepper)
- 2 jars

FODY'S LOW FODMAP MARINARA SAUCE

- 1 tsp dried parsley
- 1 tsp dried basil
- 1 tsp dried oregano
- 2 chicken breasts

- 1/4 cup rice flour
- 1 egg
- 1/2 cup bread crumbs
- 1 tsp dried parsley

INSTRUCTIONS

1. Preheat the oven to 425 F. Place all the vegetables on a baking sheet, toss with olive oil and season with salt and pepper. Place in oven and let cook 25 minutes.
2. While the vegetables are cooking, warm a large metal pot on medium high heat. Remove the sausage from the casing and place on the hot pan, let brown, about 2-3 minutes, then flip and cook on the other side. Break up into quarters then add the

Fody Low FODMAP Marinara Sauce

1. parsley, basil and oregano. Bring to a simmer and let cook.

2. Once vegetables are done, cool slightly, then blend in a blender until smooth. Add 1-2 ladles of

3. Low FODMAP Pasta Sauce

4. to loosen the vegetables, if needed. Add the cooked, pureed roasted vegetables to the tomato sauce and continue cooking. Total cook time of tomato sauce is 1 to 1 1/2 hours.

5. Meanwhile, place the flour, eggs, and breadcrumbs in different dishes. Mix the parsley with the bread crumbs and whisk the egg. Slice the chicken breasts in half, lengthwise and season with salt & pepper. Dredge in flour, then in egg, then in breadcrumbs.

6. Place on the hot baking sheet, once the vegetables are removed after roasting. Drizzle olive oil on both sides of chicken and cook 18 to 20 minutes on one side (should be browned), flip, and finish cooking 7 to 10 minutes on the other side until cooked through. Once your Low FODMAP chicken parmesan is cooked, top with a little

parmesan cheese and tomato sauce and finish in the broiler for 2 minutes.

7. Serve one piece of Low FODMAP chicken parmesan with 1/2 cup to 1 cup of pasta tossed and topped with the delicious Low FODMAP roasted vegetable sauce.

LOW FODMAP CARROT TOMATO SOUP

INGREDIENTS

- 2 tablespoons (30 ml) olive oil
- 2 teaspoons (3 g)ginger
- 1 pound (450 g) carrots, peeled and chopped into 1 inch slices
- 1.5 pounds (680 g)tomatoes
- 1 teaspoon oregano
- 1 teaspoon salt
- 2 cups (500 ml) low FODMAP vegetable stock*
- 1 bay leaf
- 2 tablespoons (15 g) nutritional yeast or grated parmesan (optional - for extra cheesiness/ use nutritional yeast for dairy free)

INSTRUCTIONS

1. In a large cooking pot, add the olive oil on a medium heat. When the oil is hot, add the ginger and carrot. Sautee a minute.
2. Add the tomatoes, oregano and salt. Stir. Add the vegetable stock, bay leaf and nutritional yeast if using. Stir until fully mixed.
3. Bring to a boil - cook for about 5 minutes, then reduce heat down to simmer. Cover and let simmer for another 20-25 minutes or until carrots are fork tender.
4. Remove the pot from the heat and fish out the bay leaf. Use an immersion blender to process until smooth. Season with salt and pepper to taste.
5. If you don't own an immersion blender you can can blend up the soup in batches using a blender. Just make sure to be careful when removing the blender lid and open away from your body.
6. Serve and enjoy!

CHICKEN TURMERIC RICE

INGREDIENTS

1. 3 tbsp olive oil OR garlic infused oil
2. 4 chicken drumsticks skinless
3. 1 tbsp turmeric
4. 1 cup | 220 gr white rice medium-grain
5. 1 large carrot finely chopped
6. 1/2 cup chickpeas canned
7. sea salt

INSTRUCTIONS

1. Heat the olive oil in a large non-stick frying pan over medium–high heat.
2. Toss in the chicken and turmeric and cook for 2–3 minutes, or until golden brown, turning often to ensure even color.
3. Cover the chicken with water and let it cook over medium heat for approx. 20 minutes, stirring occasionally.
4. Add the rice, carrot, chickpeas and cover again with water. Bring to the boil, salt to taste, then reduce the heat to low. Cover and simmer for another 15 minutes until all the water is absorbed and the rice is tender. Give everything a good stir and season to taste, if necessary.

5. Remove from the heat and stand, covered, for a further 15 minutes.

LOW FODMAP CREAMY HAM AND POTATO SOUP

CREAMY HAM POTATO SOUP

- 195 g (1 1/2 cup)   shaved ham (we used leftover Christmas ham)*
- 80 g (1 cup)   leek (green leaves only, finely chopped)*
- 800 g   potatoes (peeled & chopped in small chunks)
- 240 g (2 large)   carrots (peeled & diced)
- 2 tbsp   dairy free spread (olive oil spread or butter)*
- 1 tbsp   garlic infused oil*
- 2 tbsp   gluten free all purpose flour*
- 625 ml (2 1/2 cup)   low FODMAP chicken stock*
- 375 ml (1 1/2 cup)   low FODMAP milk*
- 6 tbsp   sweet corn kernels (frozen or fresh)
- 1 tsp   dried chives*
- Season with   salt & pepper

- 2 tsp fresh parsley (finely chopped, optional)

INSTRUCTIONS

1. Prep the ham, leek leaves, potato and carrot. Measure out the sweet corn.
2. Place a large saucepan over medium heat. Add the dairy free spread or butter and fry the leek leaves and carrot for 3 minutes until the carrot starts to soften.
3. Then add the potato, ham and garlic infused oil. Cook for 2 minutes, stirring every now and then to stop the vegetables sticking to the bottom.
4. Mix through the flour and cook for a further minute. Then pour the stock into the saucepan. Mix well and bring to the boil. Allow to cook for 12 minutes, stirring every couple of minutes, until the potatoes are tender.
5. Reduce the heat to medium-low and add the milk, sweet corn and dried chives. Stir over the heat until thickened - this will take about 5 minutes.

- Taste and season with salt and pepper if
  needed.
- Serve warm and garnish with a sprinkle of
  parsley if desired.
- If at any point your soup becomes too thick
  just stir through another splash of milk.

LOW FODMAP ENCHILADAS

INGREDIENTS

FOR THE ENCHILADA SAUCE

- 2 tbsp garlic-infused olive oil
- 2 tbsp gluten-free flour
- 500 ml (2 cups) low FODMAP broth
- 1/4 tsp ground cumin
- 1/4 tsp oregano
- 1–2 tsp chili powder*
- A pinch of salt
- 70 g (1/3 cup) tomato paste
- 200 g (7/8 cup) canned diced tomatoes
- If necessary: 1-2 tbsp corn starch to thicken
  the sauce

FOR THE ENCHILADAS

- 350 g (12 oz) Quorn vegetarian mince (you can also use minced beef)
- 2 red bell peppers
- 1/2 tsp smoked ground paprika
- 12 corn tortillas
- 200 g (1 3/4 cup) grated cheese
- FOR GARNISH
- Lactose-free sour cream or creme fraiche
- Avocado (max. 30 g per serving)
- Fresh cilantro

INSTRUCTIONS

FOR THE SAUCE

1. Heat two tablespoons of olive oil in a pan. I used garlic-infused oil to add some garlic flavor to the dish.
2. Add two tablespoons of gluten-free flour and stir through. Then add the spices and stir everything together.
3. Add the stock, tomato paste and canned tomatoes and stir everything together with a whisk. Bring the sauce to a boil. Then turn down the heat and leave the sauce to simmer for 15 minutes.

4. If you find the sauce too thin, you can add 1-
   2 tbsp corn starch to thicken it.

FOR THE FILLING

1. Heat a splash of olive oil in a pan and add
   the Quorn vegetarian mince.
2. Cut the bell pepper into pieces and add this
   to the pan too. Fry the mince and the bell
   pepper on medium high heat for about 8
   minutes.
3. Add two tablespoons of enchilada sauce to
   the minced meat and season with smoked
   ground paprika, pepper and salt. Turn off
   the heat.

PREPARING THE ENCHILADAS

1. Pre-heat the oven to 180 degrees Celsius
   (350 F)
2. Take the casserole dish and divide a few
   tablespoons of enchilada sauce over the
   bottom (a thin layer of sauce).

3. Take a corn tortilla and spread a thin layer of sauce on top. Scoop some of the vegetarian minced meat mixture on top of it and sprinkle with grated cheese.
4. Rolling up corn tortillas without them falling apart is almost impossible. Therefore, I choose to fold them in half carefully and layer them next to each other and on top of each other in the oven dish like that.
5. Pour the rest of the enchilada sauce on top of the tortillas in the oven dish and sprinkle the rest of the cheese on top.
6. Put the enchiladas in the oven for 20 minutes. Serve with lactose-free sour cream, a few slices of avocado (max. 30 gram per serving) and fresh cilantro to taste.

THE FODMAP EVERYDAY GREEN KIWI SMOOTHIE

INGREDIENTS:

- 1 cup (170 g) seedless green grapes
- 1 kiwi, peeled and cut into chunks

- 2 tablespoons water
- 8- inches (20 cm) of unpeeled English, hothouse style cucumber, cut into chunks
- 2 cups (40 g) baby spinach, (for a milder taste) or chopped stemmed, washed and dried Lacinato kale leaves (for a bolder taste) or a combo
- 1 ½ to 2 cups ice cubes

INSTRUCTIONS

1. Place all the items in blender in order listed - except the ice. Pulse on an off to begin blending, then blend on high speed until puréed, blended and smooth. Add the smaller amount of ice cubes and blend until frosty, pulsing on and off.
2. Add more ice cubes if desired. Serve immediately as it separates upon sitting. It will still be good, just not as pretty.

LOW FODMAP HERBED TUNA MELT

INGREDIENTS

- 2 low FODMAP English muffins, sliced in half (or 2 to 4 slices of low FODMAP bread, depending on recommended serving size) // notes 1 & 2
- 1 (5-ounce) can tuna packed in olive oil, drained // note 3
- ¼ cup mayonnaise, such as Hellmann's
- 2 tablespoons finely chopped fresh chives (or 2 teaspoons dried chives)
- 2 teaspoons finely chopped fresh flat-leaf parsley (or ½ teaspoon dried parsley)
- 2 teaspoon finely chopped fresh basil leaves (or ½ teaspoon dried basil)
- Sea salt and freshly cracked black pepper
- 2 tablespoons shredded cheddar cheese // note 4
- ½ medium Roma tomato, thinly sliced into 4 slices

INSTRUCTIONS

1. Move oven rack to 4-6 inches below broiler. Turn on the broiler.
2. Toast the bottom halves of the English muffins (or 2 slices of bread). Transfer the

toasted bread to an ungreased broiler-safe baking sheet or broiler pan.

3. In a small bowl, mix tuna, mayonnaise, chives, parsley, and basil. Add salt and pepper, and adjust seasonings to taste.

4. Stir in shredded cheddar cheese until well-mixed.

5. Divide the tuna mixture evenly onto the toasted bread.

6. Broil the open-faced tuna sandwiches for 5-7 minutes, or until the cheese melts and the tuna is warm. Cooking times are suggestions based on what works in my kitchen. To minimize the risk of burnt cheese, I recommend starting with less cooking time and adding time as needed.

7. Meanwhile, toast the remaining 2 English muffin halves (or 2 slices of bread).

8. Remove the tuna melts from the oven. Top each half with 2 tomato slices and a just-toasted English muffin half. Cool slightly before enjoying warm.

FODY'S LOADED SPICY CHICKEN NACHOS

INGREDIENTS:

- 1 4oz. bag LOW FODMAP gluten free tortilla chips
- 1 lb. chicken tenders
- 1 Tbsp Fody's Taco Seasoning
- 1 cup canned black beans, drained
- 1 cup grated sharp cheddar cheese
- ¼ cup queso fresco, crumbled
- ¼ cup green onion, sliced (only the green parts)
- ¾ cup cherry tomatoes, roughly chopped
- ¼ cup canned & sliced black olives, drained
- 2 Tbsp fresh cilantro, finely chopped
- ½ cup mashed avocado (2 Tbsp per person)
- ½ cup Lactose free sour cream
- ½ cup Fody's Medium Salsa

INSTRUCTIONS

1. Preheat your oven to 375 degrees and spray a baking dish with non-stick cooking spray.
2. Then place your chicken tenders in the dish and season them with your taco seasoning. Bake them for 15 minutes then use a fork and knife to shred them once done.

3. Next lower your oven to 350 degrees and line a rimmed baking sheet with parchment paper. Arrange half the tortilla chips on the pan then layer it with half your shredded chicken, black beans, green onions, tomatoes, olives and cheddar cheese. Repeat the layers with chips, chicken, beans, onion, tomatoes, olives and cheese.
4. Bake your nachos for 10-15 minutes or until the cheese has fully melted.
5. Once done, sprinkle your queso fresco and cilantro over the top and serve with your sour cream, mashed avocado and medium salsa.

NEW ORLEANS STYLE LOW FODMAP GUMBO

INGREDIENTS:

For the Roux:

- ¼ cup (60 ml) Low FODMAP Garlic-Infused Oil, preferably made with avocado oil or other neutral flavored oil; not olive oil
- 1 teaspoon asafetida; use gluten-free if following a gluten-free diet

- ¼ cup (36 g) low FODMAP gluten-free all-purpose flour

For the Gumbo:

- 2 tablespoons tomato paste
- 1 tablespoon red miso paste
- 1 cup (64 g) chopped chives
- 1 cup (104 g) diced green bell pepper
- 1 cup (72 g) finely chopped leeks, green parts only
- 1 cup (64 g) chopped scallions, green parts only
- ½ cup (38 g) chopped celery
- 3 tablespoons smoked paprika
- 1 tablespoon dried basil
- 1 tablespoon dried oregano
- 2 teaspoon dried thyme
- 1 teaspoon black pepper
- 1 teaspoon salt
- 1 teaspoon white pepper
- 1/4 teaspoon cayenne
- 1 cup (75 g) rinsed, shredded, canned jackfruit,
- 1 cup (75 g) chopped trimmed oyster mushrooms

- 20 pods (200 okra, chopped
- 3 cups (720 ml) Low FODMAP Vegetable Broth, plus extra as needed
- 1, 14.5-ounce (411 g) can fire roasted diced tomatoes
- 1 tablespoon white vinegar
- 1 teaspoon sugar
- 2 bay leaves
- 1 cup (139 g) rinsed, drained, canned butter beans
- Chopped flat-leaf parsley

Optional Additions (to taste):

- Low FODMAP hot sauce, such as Tabasco
- Low FODMAP sausage, meat, poultry, plant-based or vegan

INSTRUCTIONS

1. For the Roux: Add oil to a 10-quart (9.5 L) stock pot set over medium heat. When oil is shimmering whisk in asafetida then whisk in flour. Continue whisking for several minutes, or until the roux becomes a rich brown, milk

chocolate color. Do not leave your roux unattended or it may burn!

2. For the Gumbo: Once the roux is a rich milk chocolate color, whisk in the tomato paste, miso, chives, green peppers, leeks, scallions and celery until well combined. Continue to cook, whisking/stirring frequently until vegetables soften, about 4 minutes.

3. While the greens are softening, prepare your Cajun creole seasoning by combining smoked paprika, basil, oregano, thyme, black pepper, salt, white pepper and cayenne together in a small bowl; set aside.

4. Add jackfruit, okra, oyster mushrooms and okra to your cooked mixture, stirring in well to incorporate. Add Cajun creole seasoning to mixture and stir until everything is thoroughly combined.

5. Stir in 3-cups (720 ml) vegetable broth, the fire roasted tomatoes, white vinegar, sugar, and bay leaves. Note: you may also add sausage or plant-based sausage at this stage depending on your preference and tolerance. Gently stir in the butter beans. Cover and a adjust heat to a low simmer.

6. Simmer for 60 minutes minimum, stirring occasionally. Add additional low FODMAP broth as needed to achieve your desired gumbo consistency. More liquid will make a thinner gumbo. Taste and adjust seasoning, adding hot sauce, if you like, or offer hot sauce at the table. We like our gumbo served with rice, garnished with parsley. Leftovers can be refrigerated in an airtight container for 3 days.

LOW FODMAP INSTANT POT BEEF POT ROAST ONE-POT MEAL.

INGREDIENTS

- 2 tablespoons garlic-infused olive oil *
- 3-4 pound beef chuck roast
- 1 cup leek, dark green leaves only, finely chopped*
- 1 ½ cups low FODMAP low sodium beef broth

- 2 tablespoons tomato paste
- 1 tablespoon coconut aminos
- 1 tablespoon fresh thyme (or 1 teaspoon dried thyme)
- 1 teaspoon kosher salt, plus more for sprinkling
- ½ teaspoon black pepper, freshly-ground, plus more for sprinkling
- 4 large carrots (about 1 pound), peeled and chopped, or 1 pound baby carrots
- 1 pound red potatoes, chopped into ½-inch pieces
- 1 cup king oyster mushrooms, halved lengthwise then sliced horizontally*

INSTRUCTIONS

1. Have the leek chopped and ready before starting; the remaining vegetables can be chopped while the roast is cooking.
2. Press the "Sauté" button on your 6-quart Instant Pot, 8-quart Instant Pot, or comparable electric pressure cooker, and add garlic-infused olive oil. While the Instant Pot is heating up, dry roast well with paper

towels. Sprinkle with kosher salt and freshly-ground black pepper.

3. Once the display on the Instant Pot reads "Hot," using tongs, add roast to the pot and sear for 2 minutes on each long side and 1 minute on each short side until all sides are brown. Remove roast to a plate.

4. Add leek and sauté for 2 minutes, stirring frequently so that it does not burn.

5. Press "Cancel" on the Instant Pot. Add beef broth to deglaze the pot, wait 15 seconds, and scrape the bottom of the pot clean with a plastic spoon.

6. Add tomato paste, coconut aminos, thyme, 1 teaspoon kosher salt and ½ teaspoon black pepper to the pot and stir. Put the roast back in the pot and scrape any juices that it left behind on the plate into the pot with a spatula (leave no flavor behind!!!). Close the lid of the Instant Pot and set pressure release valve to "Sealing." Press the "Meat" button and set timer for 50 minutes. While the roast is cooking, chop carrots, potatoes and oyster mushrooms.

7. Once the cooking cycle has completed, quick release the pressure. Using a fresh set of tongs, carefully flip the roast over to the opposite side in the pot. Add the carrots, potatoes and mushrooms to the broth around the roast, being careful of hot, splashing broth. Use the tongs to gently push the vegetables as far down into the broth as possible.

8. Close the lid of the Instant Pot and set pressure release valve to "Sealing." Press the "Pressure Cook" or "Manual" button and set timer for 3 minutes.

9. Once the cooking cycle has completed, quick release the pressure. Carefully remove roast to a serving platter using tongs. Using a slotted spoon, remove vegetables to a serving vessel. Pour pan juices into a measuring cup or gravy boat and serve over the meat and potatoes.

LOW FODMAP PUMPKIN PIE

INGREDIENTS

- 1 9-inch | 28cm GF-low FODMAP pie crust OR sheet of GF-low FODMAP puffed pastry
- 21 oz | 600g japanese pumpkin (approx. 15.8oz | 450g pumpkin puree)*
- 2 eggs
- 3.5 oz | 100g brown sugar
- 2 tbsp cornstarch
- 1/2 tsp salt
- 2 heaped tsp ground cinnamon
- 1/2 tsp ground nutmeg
- 1/2 tsp ground ginger
- 3.4 oz | 100ml almond milk

INSTRUCTIONS

1. Pre-heat oven to 375ºF | 180ºC degrees. Fit the pie crust into a 4*14-inch | 35*11cm square tart pan and prick the dough all over with a fork.
2. Cut the seedless, skinless pumpkin in chunks and steam for 15 to 20 minutes or until soft. Mash with a fork and set aside to cool.
3. Beat eggs with sugar for two minutes, until bubbles form.

4. Add the pumpkin puree, cornstarch, milk, salt and spices and mix until well combined.
5. Pour the mixture in the tart pan and cook for 45 to 55 minutes, or until centre is set.
6. Remove from oven and leave to rest for 2 hours before serving.

LOW FODMAP RED VELVET CUPCAKES

INGREDIENTS

- 225 g gluten-free flour
- ¾ tsp baking soda
- 1 tsp xanthan gum
- A pinch of salt
- 200 g white sugar

- 2 tbsp cacao powder
- 85 g butter, at room temperature
- 2 eggs, at room temperature
- ½ tsp vanilla extract
- 1 tsp vinegar
- 240 ml lactose-free milk
- Red food colouring

FOR THE FROSTING

- 200 g lactose-free cream cheese, at room temperature
- 300 g powdered sugar
- 100 g butter

INSTRUCTIONS

1. Pre-heat the oven to 160 degrees Celcius.
2. Place 12 baking cups into a muffin tin.
3. Put the lactose-free milk into a bowl and add a teaspoon of vinegar. Stir together and leave for 15 minutes. Like this, you make something similar to buttermilk, but lactose-free.

4. Put the gluten-free flour, baking soda, xanthan gum, salt, sugar and cacao powder together in a bowl and stir together.
5. Add the butter, eggs, vanilla extract and a few drops of red food colouring to the flour mixture. Mix together.
6. Finally, add the milk and stir everything together. Add some more food colouring, one drop at a time, until you get the desired red colour.
7. Divide the batter over the 12 baking cups. Tap the muffin tin onto the table a few times to remove the air from the batter.
8. Bake the cupcakes in the oven for 25 minutes. The cupcakes are done when a toothpick comes out clean.
9. Leave the cupcakes to cool entirely.
10. In the meantime, make the frosting. Mix the cream cheese and the butter into a fluffy mixture. Add the powdered sugar little by little and mix it into a creamy frosting.
11. Put the frosting into a piping bag and pipe some frosting on top of every cupcake. Cream cheese frosting is softer than buttercream frosting, therefore the frosting

won't get hard like buttercream frosting
does.

12. You can store the cupcakes in a closed box
in the fridge for 2-3 days.

SKILLET LOW FODMAP SCALLION BACON CORNBREAD

INGREDIENTS:

Cornbread:

- 6 slices meaty bacon
- 1 ½ cups (228 g) medium grind cornmeal, such as Bob's Red Mill Gluten Free Medium Grind Cornmeal
- ¾ cup (109 g) low FODMAP gluten-free all-purpose flour, such as Bob's Red Mill 1 to 1 Gluten Free Baking Flour
- 2 ½ teaspoons baking powder; use gluten-free if following a gluten-free diet
- 1 teaspoon salt
- ½ teaspoon baking soda
- 1 ¼ cups (300 ml) lactose-free buttermilk
- ¼ cup (60 ml) pure maple syrup

- ¼ cup (60 ml) neutral flavor vegetable oil, such as canola
- 2 large eggs, at room temperature
- ¼ cup (16 g) chopped scallions, green parts only
- Glaze – Optional
- 1 tablespoon melted unsalted butter
- 1 tablespoon pure maple syrup

INSTRUCTIONS

1. Position rack in middle of oven. Preheat oven to 425°F (220°C).
2. Place the bacon in a 10-inch (25 cm) cast iron skillet and set over low-medium heat. Cook bacon, flipping once, until crisp. Remove bacon to paper towels to absorb excess fat. Leave 1 tablespoon bacon fat in pan; save or discard the rest. Place bacon strips back in pan.
3. Meanwhile, whisk the cornmeal, flour, baking powder, salt and baking soda together in a medium sized mixing bowl to aerate and combine.
4. In a separate bowl whisk together the lactose-free buttermilk, maple syrup, oil and

the eggs until well combined. Combine the wet and dry ingredients, then fold in the chopped scallions. Scrape into cast-iron pan over bacon and spread evenly to fill the pan.

5. Bake cornbread for about 20 to 30 minutes or until golden brown and a toothpick inserted in the center comes out clean. All to cool for about 5 minutes, then unmold, so you can see the pretty bacon. Brush with optional graze, if using. Simply stir the butter and maple syrup together and brush over the top. Serve immediately cut into 8 wedges. Skillet Low FODMAP Scallion Bacon Cornbread is best served the same day.

LOW FODMAP SPAGHETTI WITH CHICKEN AND CHERRY TOMATOES

INGREDIENTS

- 6 ounces brown rice spaghetti

- 4 small chicken breasts (or 2 larger chicken breasts cut in half butterfly-style to yield 4 pieces)
- Salt and pepper
- 2 tablespoons avocado oil
- ¾ cup dry white wine (I used Pinot Grigio)
- 12 (or up to 180 grams) cherry tomatoes // see note
- 2 tablespoons butter
- 1 tablespoon garlic-infused olive oil
- 2 teaspoons dried basil (I like Litehouse Freeze Dried Basil)
- Optional garnish: Thinly sliced fresh basil

INSTRUCTIONS

1. Cook spaghetti according to package instructions. Turn off the heat. Carefully reserve ¼ cup pasta water and set aside for later. Drain the cooked spaghetti and return the pasta to the pot. Toss with a bit of olive oil to help prevent the spaghetti from sticking.

2. Meanwhile, season chicken with salt and pepper. Heat the avocado oil in a large skillet (with a lid) over medium to medium-

high heat. Once hot, add the chicken, cover, and cook for 5 minutes without disturbing. Flip, re-cover, and cook for another 5 to 7 minutes, or until fully cooked. Chicken is considered fully cooked when a food thermometer inserted into the thickest part reads 165°F. Transfer cooked chicken to a clean cutting board to cool slightly. Slice the chicken into bite-sized pieces. I like to do this while the tomatoes are simmering.

3. To the now-empty skillet, add the wine and cherry tomatoes. Simmer for 10 minutes, or until the tomatoes start to soften. Using a fork or flat-edged spatula, carefully burst the tomatoes. Continue cooking for 1-2 minutes.

4. Reduce heat to medium. Add the butter, garlic-infused olive oil, dried basil, and ¼ cup reserved pasta water to the tomato-wine sauce. Continue to cook until the butter has melted and the sauce thickens slightly. Turn off the heat. Season with salt and pepper.

5. Add the chicken and cooked spaghetti to the sauce. Toss to mix.

6. Serve warm topped with an optional sprinkle of thinly sliced basil.

GREEN BEANS & BACON

INGREDIENTS

- 80 g bacon strips (diced)*
- 1 tbsp garlic infused oil*
- 280 g green beans
- 4 tbsp green onions/scallions (green leaves only, finely sliced)*
- Season with salt & pepper
- 1 1/2 tbsp pumpkin seeds (lightly toasted)*
- small lemon (cut into wedges)

INSTRUCTIONS

1. Trim the ends off the green beans. Finely sliced the green leaves of the spring onion/scallions. Dice the bacon.
2. Place a large frypan over medium high heat. Before you add any oil, toast the pumpkin seeds. Place the pumpkin seeds in the frypan and toast until lightly golden. Then remove from the pan and place in a bowl to cool.
3. Place the frypan back over the heat. Add the garlic infused oil and bacon. Fry the bacon

bits until crispy. Remove the from the pan and place on a paper towel-lined plate.

4. Return the frypan to the heat and add the green beans and spring onion. Fry for 2 to 3 minutes until the green beans are tender and slightly golden.

5. Transfer to a platter. Season generously with black pepper and a squeeze of lemon juice. Roughly chop the pumpkin seeds. Top the platter with the chopped pumpkin seeds, crispy bacon and extra lemon wedges. Serve warm.

ROASTED SWEET POTATO, QUINOA AND FRIED EGG LUNCH BOWL

INGREDIENTS

- Half a medium sweet potato, cut into cubes
  - o tsp smoked paprika

- 1 tsp olive oil
- 1/2 cup quinoa uncooked
- 1 cup Low FODMAP vegetable or chicken stock
- 4 eggs
- 1 tbsp butter
- Salt and pepper to taste

INSTRUCTIONS

1. Preheat the oven to 200C. Line a tray with baking paper and toss the sweet potato cubes with the smoked paprika and olive oil. Roast for 25 minutes or until golden brown.
2. In the meantime, place quinoa into a small saucepan with the stock (or water) over medium heat. Bring to a boil, then lower heat and simmer until cooked through (approx. 15 minutes)
3. In a large fry pan, melt the butter over medium heat. Crack eggs into the pan one at a time and cook for approximately 3 minutes, or until white is completely set. Remove from the heat and set aside

4. Divide the quinoa and sweet potato into 2 bowls and stir to combine. Add eggs on top and season with salt and pepper to taste.

CHICKEN MADRAS CURRY

INGREDIENTS

- 2 tbs olive oil
- 2 tbs garlic infused olive oil
- 37 g tsp cinnamon
- 1 tbs ginger, finely chopped
- 1 tsp turmeric
- 1 tsp cumin seeds
- 1 tsp ground coriander
- 1 tsp garam masala
- 1/2 tsp cayenne pepper
- Chicken thigh fillets, cut in half
- 8 fresh curry leaves medium tomatoes, roughly chopped
- 1/3 cup coconut milk, canned
- 1/4 cup coriander, roughly chopped

INSTRUCTIONS

1. Heat the regular olive oil in a large saucepan over medium heat. Place the ginger and

cinnamon in the pan and cook for 1 minute.
Add in the garlic infused olive oil, turmeric,
cumin, ground coriander, garam masala,
cayenne and curry leaves. Cook for 5
minutes, stirring constantly.

2. Add the chicken thighs to coat, and cook for
3 minutes. Stir in the roughly chopped
tomatoes and cook for 15 minutes.

3. Add the coconut milk and stir, simmer for 1-
2 minutes, then remove from heat.

RICE PAPER ROLLS WITH PEANUT DIPPING SAUCE

INGREDIENTS

- Dried vermicelli noodles
- Firm tofu
- 2 tbsp sesame oil
- 2 tbsp cornstarch

- o large carrot, grated
- 1/2 a cucumber, thinly sliced
- 1 cup red cabbage
- 1/4 cup coriander leaves
- 8 rice paper wrappers
- 1/3 cup peanut butter
  - o tbsp rice wine vinegar
- 1 tbsp maple syrup
  - o tbsp soy sauce
- 1 tbsp sesame oil
- 2 to 3 tbsp water, as needed

INSTRUCTIONS

1. Place vermicelli noodles into a bowl and cover with boiling water. Let stand until the noodles are soft and then drain. Cut noodles into short lengths with kitchen

2. Meanwhile, heat 2 tbsp sesame oil in a fry pan over medium heat and slice tofu into small rectangles. Toss the tofu in the cornstarch and add to the fry pan, flipping on all sides until evenly browned, approximately 5 minutes. Remove from the pan and set aside.

3. Soak rice paper wrappers in cold water until soft and pliable.
4. Add a small handful of vermicelli noodles and layer carrot, cucumber, red cabbage, coriander and tofu on top. Gently roll over once, tuck in the edges, and continue rolling until the seam is sealed.
5. Repeat with remaining wrappers, noodles, vegetables and tofu
6. To make the dipping sauce, whisk together the peanut butter, rice vinegar, soy sauce, maple syrup and sesame oil. Whisk in 2 - 3 tbsp of water as needed to make a smooth, creamy sauce
7. Serve rice paper rolls with dipping sauce

CHOCOLATE WATTLESEED SELF-SAUCING PUDDING

INGREDIENTS

- 2 tbs wattleseeds*
  - cup gluten-free flour
- 3/4 cup caster sugar
- 1/2 cup cocoa powder
- 1/2 cup low FODMAP milk of your choice

- 1 tsp vanilla essence
- 1.5 tbs butter, melted
- 1/2 cup brown sugar
- 1 3/4 cups boiling water

INSTRUCTIONS

1. Preheat an oven to 180°C/356°F and prepare either an 8 cup capacity ovenproof dish or 6 x 150ml ramekins by lightly greasing with oil or butter. Soak wattleseeds in boiling water for 20 minutes, then drain.
2. In a medium-size bowl, combine the flour, caster sugar and 2 tbs of the cocoa powder. Add milk, vanilla, wattleseeds and melted butter - stir to combine. Pour the mixture into the prepared pan or evenly into each ramekin. Use a spoon or spatula to smooth over.
3. In a small bowl, mix together the remaining cocoa and brown sugar. Sift this over the prepared pan or ramekin with the mixture in it. Top the pudding with boiling water.
4. Bake for 30-35 minutes or until the top is firm. Stand for approximately 10 minutes

before serving to cool slightly. Dust with cocoa powder and serve immediately.

PARMESAN & THYME ROASTED PARSNIPS

INGREDIENTS

- 6 tbsp polenta (cornmeal)
- Parmesan, grated
- tbsp thyme leaves
- 2kg Parsnips, quartered and core removed
- 6 tbsp olive oil
- Parsley, roughly chopped

INSTRUCTIONS

1. Preheat the oven to 220C/430F
2. Combine the polenta, parmesan and thyme in a large bowl, and set aside.
3. Bring a pot of salted water to the boil, add the parsnips and cook for 6 mins or until just tender. Drain.
4. While parsnips are still hot, toss in the parmesan mixture to coat.

5. Set a roasting tin over the stove top and heat up the olive oil. Add the parsnips and coat in the oil.
6. Move the tin to the oven and roast for 30 mins, turning halfway through
7. Sprinkle with parsley and serve

CRANBERRY SAUCE

INGREDIENTS

- Fresh or frozen cranberries
- cup of sugar
- 1 cup of water
- 1/4 tsp cinnamon
- Pinch of nutmeg

INSTRUCTIONS

1. Add the water and sugar into a saucepan on medium-high heat and bring to a boil. Stir until the sugar is dissolved.
2. Add the cranberries to the saucepan and bring to a boil.
3. Turn the heat to low and simmer for 5-10 minutes until the majority of cranberries have burst.

4. Remove from heat and mix in the cinnamon and nutmeg

5. Let the sauce cool completely, then transfer to a bowl and store in the refrigerator until ready to serve.

BLUEBERRY POPSICLES

INGREDIENTS

- 2 cups lactose-free yoghurt
- cup lactose-free milk
- cups blueberries (fresh or frozen)
- 1 tsp cinnamon
- 1 tbs maple syrup
- 1/2 tsp vanilla essence

INSTRUCTIONS

1. Place all ingredients in a blender and blend until smooth

2. Pour the mixture into popsicle/icy pole moulds, insert sticks and freeze for approximately 4 hours or until set.

WOOD-FIRED LOW FODMAP HOT HONEY CHICKEN WINGS

INGREDIENTS:

Marinade:

- 1 tablespoon Low FODMAP Garlic-Infused Oil, made with vegetable oil, or purchased equivalent
- 1 teaspoon low FODMAP onion powder, such as FreeFod or Fodmazing
- 1 teaspoon Worcestershire sauce
- ½ teaspoon smoked paprika
- 3- pounds (1.4 kg) chicken wings, flats and drumettes
- Kosher salt
- Freshly ground black pepper

Hot Honey Glaze:

- 2 tablespoons rice vinegar or apple cider vinegar
- 2 tablespoons Worcestershire sauce
- 1 teaspoon low FODMAP garlic powder, such as FreeFod or Fodmazing
- ½ cup (113 g; 1 stick) unsalted butter, melted
- ½ cup (120 ml) Sriracha
- 2 tablespoons honey

INSTRUCTIONS

1. For The Marinade: In a large mixing bowl whisk together the Low FODMAP Garlic-Infused Oil, low FODMAP onion powder, Worcestershire sauce and smoked paprika. Add the chicken wings and toss the coat. Season liberally with salt and pepper and toss again. Let wings marinate while you tend to your oven.
2. Preheat your outdoor oven with hardwood to about 500°F (260°C); we used an Ooni Karu 16 Multi-Fuel Pizza Oven. Have ready a cast-iron pan that can hold all of the wings, such as a 12-inch (30.5 cm) skillet. Make sure entire skillet, including handle, can fit in the oven with the door closed.
3. Scrape wings and marinade into cast-iron skillet. Place in center of oven, close door, and roast for 15 minutes. Meanwhile, make your glaze.
4. For the Glaze: In a small mixing bowl, whisk together the vinegar, Worcestershire sauce and low FODMAP garlic powder until powder dissolves. Whisk in the melted

butter, Sriracha and honey until glaze
ingredients are well combined.

5. After 15 minutes of cooking, remove the
    wings from the oven, flip them all over using
    tongs, and brush or spoon over about half of
    the glaze. Return to oven and roast 10
    minutes more, top with remaining glaze,
    and then cook for 5 more minutes.

6. Get ready to eat the best wings ever! Pass
    the napkins.

VEGAN LOW FODMAP CORNBREAD

INGREDIENTS:

- 1 ¼ cups (300 ml) unsweetened almond milk
- 1 tablespoon lemon juice
- 2 tablespoons warm water
- 1 ½ teaspoons Ener-G Egg Replacer
- 1 ¼ cups (173 g) fine-ground cornmeal, such
  as Indian Head Old Fashioned Stone Ground
  Yellow Corn Meal

- 1 cup (145 g) low FODMAP gluten-free al-purpose flour, such as Bob's Red Mill 1 to 1 Gluten Free Baking Flour
- 1/3 cup (65 g) sugar
- 2 teaspoons baking powder; use gluten-free if following a gluten-free diet
- ¾ teaspoon salt
- ½ teaspoon baking soda
- ¼ cup (57 g) melted butter replacement, such as Earth Balance Vegan Buttery Sticks, cooled

INSTRUCTIONS

1. Position rack in middle of oven. Preheat oven to 400°F (200°C). Coat an 8-inch by 8-inch (20 cm by 20 cm) square metal baking pan with nonstick spray.
2. Measure out your almond milk and whisk in the lemon juice; set aside for 5 minutes. In a small bowl, whisk together the warm water and Ener-G Egg Replacer; set aside as well.
3. Add the cornmeal, flour, sugar, baking powder, salt and baking soda to a large mixing bowl; whisk to combine. In a

separate bowl whisk together the soured alt milk, vegan "egg" and the melted buttery margarine. Add the wet mixture to the dry and whisk just until combined.

4. Scrape cornbread batter into the prepared pan and smooth the top, if needed, into an even layer.

5. Bake for about 20 to 25 minutes, until a toothpick comes out clean. Place pan on wire rack and allow to cool for about 5 minutes – but do try it warm if you can time it right! Cut into 16 servings (4 by 4 grid) and serve. Cornbread can be stored in an airtight container, once cooled, at room temperature for up to 2 days. It also freezes well for up to a month. Just wrap up thoroughly in plastic wrap and then slip into a zip top bag.

LOW FODMAP HONEY LEMON PAN ROASTED CARROTS

INGREDIENTS:

- 1- pound (455 g) trimmed, peeled slender carrots, cut into 4 to 6-inch (10 cm to 15 cm) lengths, halved lengthwise
- 2 tablespoons unsalted butter
- 1 tablespoon honey
- 1 tablespoon rice syrup
- 1 tablespoon freshly squeezed lemon juice
- Kosher salt
- Freshly ground black pepper
- Chopped flat-leaf parsley; optional

INSTRUCTIONS

1. Choose a wide sauté pan that will generously accommodate the amount of carrots. Fill with a couple of inches of water and bring to a simmer over medium heat. Add carrots and cook for a few minutes or until just tender when pierced with a sharp knife. Drain well.

2. Wipe out the pan and return to the stove over low heat and add the butter, honey, and rice syrup. Stir together and cook until the butter melts, then add the lemon juice and the carrots, tossing well to coat. Turn heat up a bit and cook the carrots, turning

them over now and then, until they are crisp tender and have some char marks here and there. Season well with salt and pepper and toss one more time, then transfer to your serving dish or individual plates and serve immediately. Sprinkle with optional parsley if you like.

LOW FODMAP CREAMED SPINACH

INGREDIENTS:

- 3- pounds (1.4 kg) well washed and NOT dried spinach – leave water clinging; we suggest young "English" style leaves
- 2 tablespoons unsalted butter
- 2 tablespoons Low FODMAP Garlic-Infused Oil, made with olive oil, or purchased equivalent

- ¾ cup (180 ml) heavy cream, lactose-free if possible
- ½ teaspoon freshly grated nutmeg
- ¼ cup (25 g) grated Parmesan
- ½ teaspoon low FODMAP garlic powder, such as FreeFod or Fodmazing
- Kosher salt
- Freshly ground black pepper

INSTRUCTIONS

1. Choose a large skillet or sauté pan that will hold all of the spinach, which is voluminous. Heat the butter and oil in the skillet over medium heat until butter melts, then add the spinach. Cook, tossing frequently (I find tongs helpful), until the spinach is cooked and wilted down. Scrape all the spinach and any juices into a colander and press as much liquid out of the spinach as possible. Use the back of a sturdy wooden spoon and truly press as hard as you can. The drier you get

the spinach at this point, the better. At this point you can chop the spinach, if you like. I often don't bother.

2. Heat the same skillet again over medium heat and add the cream and nutmeg; whisk the spice in. Bring to a simmer and cook until it reduces a bit, about 5 minutes. Add the spinach, parmesan, and low FODMAP garlic powder, season with salt and pepper, toss well and cook until the spinach heated through, about 5 more minutes. Serve immediately.

LOW FODMAP VIENNESE FARMER CHEESE CAKE

INGREDIENTS:

Pastry Crust:

- ¾ cup (109 g) plus 2 tablespoons low FODMAP gluten-free all-purpose flour, such as Bob's Red Mill 1 to 1 Gluten Free Baking Flour
- ¼ cup (50 g) sugar
- ¼ teaspoon xanthan gum

- Pinch salt
- 7 tablespoons (99 g) unsalted butter, at cool room temperature, cut into small pieces, plus extra
- 2 large egg yolks; save 1 egg white for the filling
- Grated zest of ½ lemon
- Grated zest of ½ orange; optional
- ¼ teaspoon vanilla extract

Cheese Cake Filling:

- 1- pound (455 g) farmer cheese, such as Friendship brand, at room temperature
- 1 cup (240 g) lactose-free sour cream, at room temperature
- ¾ cup (149 g) sugar, divided
- ¼ cup (60 ml) lactose-free whole milk; at room temperature, optional
- 2 tablespoons cornstarch
- 2 teaspoons vanilla extract
- Grated zest of ½ lemon
- Grated zest of ½ orange; optional
- ¼ teaspoon salt

- 4 large eggs; separated, plus 1 large egg white (saved from crust), at room temperature
- ¼ cup (22 g) sliced blanched almonds
- ¼ cup (52 g) plump raisins; plumped with 1 ½ tablespoons Grand Marnier as an option

INSTRUCTIONS

1. For the Crust: Combine the flour, sugar, xanthan gum and salt in stand mixer bowl. Using the flat paddle attachment, add 7 tablespoons butter and mix on low-medium speed until the mixture resembles coarse crumbs. Whisk together the egg yolks, lemon zest, orange zest if using, and the vanilla extract and add to the dry mixture. Mix until the dough is evenly moistened and holds together when pressed between your fingers. Gather together by hand, knead it a couple of times, press into a flat disc and wrap with plastic wrap. Refrigerate for about 30 minutes. You can also make this dough this by hand with a pastry-blender. If you are short on time, I have successfully

patted it into the prepped pan right away, with well-floured fingertips.

2. Position rack in lower third of oven. Preheat to 400°F (200°C). Line the bottom of a 9-inch (23 cm) springform pan with parchment paper as follows: Cut a piece of parchment larger than the pan's bottom and place on top of pan bottom. Attach the springform sides so that they go over the paper and seal it into place as you snap the springform shut. The paper will overhang the exterior of the pan; that's what you want. This will allow you to remove the cake from the pan bottom easily, to place on your serving platter.

3. Lightly butter the insides of the pan, both the parchment and pan's sides. Press the dough firmly and evenly into the pan, bringing the dough about 1-inch (2.5 cm) up the sides. Pierce the dough all over with a fork and freeze for 10 minutes.

4. Bake for about 10 to 12 minutes or until the crust is just beginning to brown. Place on a wire rack and cool completely.

5. For the Filling: Place the farmer cheese into your stand mixer bowl, fitted with flat paddle attachment. Beat on medium speed for about 30 seconds; you want to smooth it out a bit. Add the sour cream, ¼ cup (50 g) of the sugar, milk (if using), cornstarch, vanilla, lemon zest, orange zest (if using), and salt and beat on low-medium speed until combined. Beat in the 4 egg yolks, one at a time; do not overmix. You want the batter to blended, but not to incorporate too much air, which could lead to excess expansion during baking, subsequent deflation and more chances of cracks forming.

6. Place egg whites in a clean, grease-free mixer bowl and beat with balloon whisk attachment on high speed until soft peaks form. Gradually add remaining ½ cup (99 g) of the sugar and beat until the egg whites form stiff, shiny peaks. Stir about a quarter of the whites into the cheese cake mixture to lighten, then fold in the rest. Pour the filling into the cooled crust and even out the top with a small offset spatula. Sprinkle the

raisins (drained of any liquid) and almonds evenly over the top.

7. Bake for 10 minutes at 400°F (200°C), then reduce the oven temperature to 350°F (180°C) and bake for about 20 to 30 minutes more or until the edges of the filling are gently puffed and barely tinged with golden brown. The center will still be wobbly; it will firm up upon cooling. Do not overbake, which might encourage cracking.

8. Remove from the oven and place on a cooling to and cool completely. Cover the top with plastic wrap and refrigerate overnight or up to 2 days. To unmold, run a small, straight icing spatula under warm water and use it to completely separate the cake from the pan, pressing out towards the pan; remove springform sides. Now take a cake lifter, loose bottom tart pan bottom or broad flat spatula and separate the pastry crust from the parchment; lift cake up and away from parchment, peel away parchment, and place cake on serving platter. Serve the cake chilled, using a hot, wet knife to slice the cake into 14 wedges.

LOW FODMAP CHOCOLATE PUDDING CAKE

INGREDIENTS:

- ¾ cup (109 g) low FODMAP gluten-free all-purpose flour, such as Bob's Red Mill 1 to 1 Gluten Free Baking Flour
- ½ cup (43 g) sifted natural cocoa powder, divided
- ½ cup (99 g) sugar
- 1 ½ teaspoons baking powder; use gluten-free if following a gluten-free diet
- ½ teaspoon salt
- ½ cup (120 ml) lactose-free whole milk, at room temperature
- 3 tablespoons neutral vegetable oil, such as canola or vegetable
- ½ cup (107 g) firmly packed light brown sugar
- ¼ teaspoon instant espresso powder; optional
- 2- ounces (55 g) semisweet or bittersweet chocolate chips or chopped chocolate
- 1 ¼ cups (300 ml) boiling water

1. Position rack in middle of oven. Preheat oven to 350°F (180°C). Have ready a 9 ½-inch by 1 ½-inch (23 cm by 4 cm) ovenproof glass or ceramic pie plate set on an aluminum foil or parchment paper lined half-sheet pan.

2. In a small bowl gently whisk together the flour, ¼ cup (21 g) of the cocoa, sugar, baking powder and salt. (You can do this right in your deep-dish pie plate, but it can make a mess. Go for it if you are neat – or daring).

3. Gently whisk the milk and oil into the dry mixture until combined; mixture will be thick. Scrape into your deep-dish pie plate if not in there already; smooth the top with a small offset spatula.

4. In a clean small bowl whisk together the brown sugar, remaining cocoa, and espresso powder, if using. Sprinkle this mixture over the top of your batter in the pie pan, then sprinkle chocolate evenly over all. Very slowly pour the boiling water evenly over pudding cake mixture, but do not stir.

5. Bake for about 30 minutes until the surface appears dry, but you do not want it baked dry all the way through. If you were to test with a toothpick, just insert the toothpick in the top ¼-inch (6 mm), not all the way down; that's where all the gooey fudgy pudding resides! The toothpick in the top section will test clean. Allow to sit for about 3 minutes before serving. Delicious served with a scoop of ice cream, or a dollop of whipped cream.

LOW FODMAP SLOW COOKED ASIAN-STYLE PORK

INGREDIENTS:

- 3- pounds (1.4 kg) trimmed pork shoulder or Boston butt (trimmed of excess fat)
- 1 ¼ teaspoons Chinese five-spice powder
- ½ teaspoon kosher salt
- ¼ teaspoon freshly ground black pepper
- 2 ½ cups (600 ml) Low FODMAP Chicken Stock, homemade or purchased equivalent

- 1 cup (240 ml) low-sodium, gluten-free soy sauce, such as San J
- ½ cup (30 g) roughly chopped scallions, green parts only
- ¼ cup (54 g) firmly packed light brown sugar
- ½ teaspoon crushed red pepper
- 1 1/2- inch (4 cm) knob peeled fresh ginger, sliced into hunks
- 1- ounce (30 g) dried shiitake mushrooms; optional
- 2 teaspoons FreeFod Garlic Replacer
- 2 tablespoons toasted sesame oil

INSTRUCTIONS

1. Use your hands to rub the pork all over with the five-spice powder, salt and pepper. Add the chicken stock, soy sauce, scallion greens, brown sugar, red pepper and ginger to your 6-quart (5.7 L) slow cooker. If you are going to use the mushrooms, crumble them into the pot now. Sprinkle the FreeFod Garlic Replacer into the liquid and stir everything together, then stir in the toasted sesame oil.
2. Add the pork, turning it over a few times to coat evenly with the liquid mixture. Cover

the cooker, set it to high, and cook for 4 hours. Check the pork; it should be tender and shred-able with a fork. If it is not, set the slow cooker to low and continue to cook until the meat is very tender, maybe another 30 minutes to an hour.

3. Transfer the pork to a cutting board, cover lightly with foil, and let rest 15 minutes. Meanwhile, pour the cooking liquid into a measuring cup and skim off and discard any fat that rises to the surface. Fish out and discard the ginger chunks but leave the scallion greens and mushrooms (if used) in there. If you like, you can boil the sauce in a pot on the stovetop to reduce a bit.

4. Shred the meat while still warm using two forks and return to the sauce. We love this dish with low FODMAP noodles, but it goes well with rice as well. A green veggie on the side such as broccoli, green beans or bok choy is a nice addition. Serve immediately or leftovers can be refrigerated in an airtight container for 4 days.

LOW FODMAP PEANUT BUTTER & JAM HEARTS

INGREDIENTS:

- ½ cup (113 g; 1 stick) unsalted butter, room temperature, cut into pieces
- ½ cup (99 g) sugar
- ½ cup (107 g) firmly packed light brown sugar
- 1 cup (258 g) no-stir style creamy peanut butter, such as Skippy brand
- ½ teaspoon vanilla extract
- 1 large egg, at room temperature
- 1 1/3 cups (194 g) low FODMAP gluten-free all-purpose flour, such as Bob's Red Mill 1 to 1 Gluten Free Baking Flour
- ¼ teaspoon salt
- 2/3 cup (211 g) strawberry or raspberry jam

INSTRUCTIONS

1. Beat the butter and sugars together in stand mixer bowl fitted with flat paddle attachment on medium speed, or in bowl with electric mixer, until well mixed and

creamy. Beat in peanut butter and vanilla until incorporated, then beat in egg.

2. Beat in flour and salt, first at low speed, then increase speed until dough forms. Cover bowl with plastic wrap and refrigerate for 15 minutes.

3. Line two half-sheet pans with parchment paper.

4. Use a scoop to portion out balls of dough about walnut size, roll them into rounds and place them evenly spaced on pans. Gently flatten the balls with your palm (flour it if necessary) to about 1/2-inch (12 mm) thickness. Create heart shapes in dough using fingertips, the end of a wooden dowel or even a small demitasse spoon. You can also simply press and created round impressions. Refrigerate while oven preheats.

5. Position racks in upper and lower third of oven. Preheat oven to 350°F (180°C). While oven preheats, stir the jam to loosen it up a bit.

6. Bake cookies for 6 minutes, then switch pans from to back and from upper to lower

rack. Bake 6 minutes more. Remove from oven and re-press and detail the heart shapes. Use a small spoon to fill the heart shaped (or round) indentations with jam. Return to oven and back for about 5 minutes more, switch pans front to back and up from down once again and bake for about another 5 minutes or until they are dry and just firm to the touch, but still a tad soft if pressed. Do not overbake. They will firm up upon cooling.

LOW FODMAP TEXAS SHEET CAKE

INGREDIENTS:

Chocolate Cake:

- 1 ¾ cups (254 g) low FODMAP gluten-free all-purpose flour, such as Bob's Red Mill 1 to 1 Gluten Free Baking Flour, plus extra for pan
- 2 cups (396 g) sugar
- 1 teaspoon baking soda

- ¼ teaspoon salt
- 1/3 cup (28 g) sifted natural cocoa
- 1 cup (226 g; 2 sticks) unsalted butter
- 1 cup (240 ml) boiling water
- 1/2 cup (120 ml) "faux" buttermilk
- 2 large eggs, at room temperature
- 1 teaspoon vanilla extract
- Icing:
- ½ cup plus 2 tablespoons (151 g) unsalted butter, at room temperature, cut into pieces
- ¼ cup (21 g) sifted natural cocoa
- 1/3 cup (75 ml) heavy cream, conventional or lactose-free
- 1 teaspoon vanilla extract
- 2 ½ cups (115 g) sifted confectioners' sugar
- 3/4 cup (100 g) finely chopped pecans or walnuts

INSTRUCTIONS

1. For The Cake: Place rack in the upper third of the oven and preheat oven to 350°F (180°C). Coat a half-sheet pan with nonstick spray, then coat with flour.

2. In a medium mixing bowl, whisk together 1 ¾ cups (254 g) flour, sugar, salt, and baking soda; set aside.

3. In a small saucepan, melt butter, then whisk in cocoa. Whisk in boiling water and allow mixture to boil for 30 seconds, then remove from heat. Pour warm chocolate over flour mixture and stir in to combine.

4. In a large liquid measuring cup whisk together the buttermilk, eggs, and vanilla. Stir this buttermilk mixture into chocolate/flour mixture until well blended. Pour into prepared pan and spread into an even layer if necessary.

5. Bake for about 20 minutes or until a toothpick inserted in the center shows a few moist crumbs. Place on rack.

6. For The Icing: As soon as the cake is pulled out of the oven, melt butter in a saucepan. Whisk in cocoa until smooth, then remove from heat. Whisk in cream, vanilla, and confectioners' sugar until smooth. Stir in nuts. Immediately pour the warm frosting over the warm cake, using a small offset spatula to help it to into the corners and

cover the cake completely. Allow to cool for at least 30 minutes to firm up icing. Cut into squares and enjoy! Cake is best served the day it is made but may be covered with plastic wrap and/or foil and stored overnight at room temperature.

LOW FODMAP TOFU BÁNH MÌ

INGREDIENTS:

For Pickled Veggies:

- 1/2 cup (75 g) long matchsticks of peeled daikon radish
- 1/2 cup (75 g) long matchsticks of hothouse cucumber (no need to peel)
- 1/2 cup (75 g) long matchsticks of peeled carrots

- 1/4 cup (60 ml) water
- 1 tablespoon rice wine vinegar
- 1 tablespoon sugar

For Tofu:

- 7- ounces (200 g) firm or extra-firm tofu, drained
- 1 teaspoon minced fresh ginger root
- 1 teaspoon toasted sesame oil
- 1/2 teaspoon soy sauce
- 1 tablespoon avocado oil or other neutral flavored oil
- 1/4 teaspoon asafetida

For Banh Mi Sauce:

- ¼ cup (80 g) low-fat mayonnaise
- 2 teaspoons fish sauce
- 2 teaspoons sriracha
- 1 teaspoon minced fresh ginger root
- 1 teaspoon fresh lemongrass paste
- 1 teaspoon lime juice
- 1 teaspoon soy sauce
- 1 teaspoon sugar

For Sandwich + Toppings:

- 6- inch (15 cm) low fodmap baguette
- 1/4 cup (4 g) cilantro sprigs
- 1 tablespoon fresh jalapeno slices

INSTRUCTIONS

1. Prepare your quick pickled vegetables: Combine the cucumbers, carrots, daikon radish, water, rice wine vinegar, and sugar in a small glass jar or plastic container. Mix well, cover, and store in room temperature for the duration of the cooking time. (You can refrigerate any extra and save for another week!)

2. Prep your tofu by wrapping it with a dry paper towel or cheese cloth and gently pressing down on it to remove excess moisture. Cut the tofu into the desired shape for your sandwich – 3-inch-long (7.5 cm) strips work well for this recipe. Set aside.

3. In a medium mixing bowl, make your tofu marinade by combining fresh ginger root, sesame oil and soy sauce. Mix well. Gently

fold in tofu strips to the marinade until each piece is well-coated.

4. Heat a medium-sized frying pan over medium heat and add avocado oil; heat until oil shimmers. Add the asafetida and allow it to toast on the pan until aromatic – about 30 seconds. Add marinated tofu pieces to your pan. Be mindful not to overcrowd and ensure that each piece lies flat with direct contact on the hot pan – this is how we get that crispy on the outside, soft on the inside texture!

5. While your tofu cooks, prep your Banh Mi sauce by mixing the mayonnaise, fish sauce, sriracha, ginger, lemongrass, lime juice, soy sauce and sugar in a small, clean mixing bowl. Whisk well and set aside.

6. Return to your pan and one-by-one, flip each marinaded tofu strip to that both sizes become crispy, golden brown. It will take about 5 minutes to brown each side, for a total of 10 minutes.

7. While your tofu finishes browning on the second side, prep your sandwich bread and garnish. Cut your low FODMAP baguette of

choice to 6-inches (15 cm) in length (optional: toast in the oven at 375°F /190°C for 10 minutes to warm it up!).

8. Once your tofu has browned on both sides, remove it from heat. Add the cooked tofu strips to your Banh Mi sauce mixture, and gently fold together until the strips are well-coated.

9. Now it's time to assemble your sandwich! Open your baguette (or low FODMAP bread of choice) and add cooked and coated tofu. Add your desired amounts of pickled vegetables, cilantro and jalapeno, slice in half to make two sandwiches and enjoy!

CONCLUSION

The LowFod Map Cookbook is a great resource for anyone looking to make healthier and more nutritious meals. It provides an easy-to-follow approach to cooking that is both nutritious and delicious. The cookbook is organized in a way that makes it easy to find the recipes that fit your lifestyle. It features a variety of recipes that are low in fat, cholesterol, and sodium, while also providing plenty of options for vegetarian and vegan meals. Overall, the LowFod Map Cookbook is a great resource for anyone interested in making healthier and more nutritious meals. It provides simple and delicious recipes to make sure that you get the most out of your meals. With its easy-to-follow approach and helpful tips, it makes it easy to create meals that are both nutritious and delicious. Whether you're looking to reduce your fat and cholesterol intake or just want to make healthier meals, the LowFod Map Cookbook is a great resource to help you do just that.

www.ingramcontent.com/pod-product-compliance
Lightning Source LLC
Chambersburg PA
CBHW050738260726
48661CB00001B/296